ENDOCRINOLOGY PEARLS

A Comprehensive Clinical Guide

Dr Essam Abdelhakim

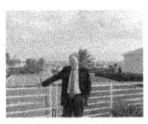

Copyright © 2024 Dr Essam Abdelhakim

All rights reserved

The characters and events portrayed in this book are fictitious. Any similarity to real persons, living or dead, is coincidental and not intended by the author.

No part of this book may be reproduced, or stored in a retrieval system, or transmitted in any form or by any means, electronic, mechanical, photocopying, recording, or otherwise, without express written permission of the publisher.

Cover design by: Art Painter
Library of Congress Control Number: 2018675309
Printed in the United States of America

CONTENTS

Title Page
Copyright
Introduction
Disclosure
Section 1: Diabetes Mellitus — 1
Section 2: Thyroid Disorders — 9
Section 3: Adrenal Disorders — 17
Section 5: Calcium and Bone Disorders — 27
Section 6: Miscellaneous Hormonal Disorders — 34
50 Questions on Endocrinology — 41

INTRODUCTION

This book provides detailed insights into a broad range of endocrine disorders, focusing on **clinical pearls, evidence-based guidelines**, and **real-world case scenarios**.

Each chapter is structured to deliver actionable knowledge, making it an ideal companion for daily clinical practice, exam preparation, and continuous professional development.

Structure of the Book

The book is organized into sections that cover key endocrine conditions, with a particular emphasis on practical, case-based approaches.

Each section focuses on **important clinical pearls** *related to common and rare endocrine disorders, diagnostic strategies, treatment options, and emerging therapies.*

The structure of each chapter is consistent, ensuring clarity and ease of use for the reader.

DISCLOSURE

Disclosure

This book has been created with the assistance of *Artificial Intelligence (AI) tools* and thoroughly reviewed and edited by the author to ensure clarity, relevance, and educational value.

While every effort has been made to provide accurate and up-to-date information, this content is intended solely for educational and informational purposes.

The author is a medical professional; however, the information provided in this book *is not a substitute for professional medical advice, diagnosis, or treatment.*

Readers are strongly advised to consult licensed healthcare providers or specialists for any medical concerns or conditions.

By using this book, **you acknowledge and agree** that the author shall not be held responsible or liable for any loss, damage, or harm whether physical, emotional, financial, or otherwise that may occur *as a result of the use or misuse of the information presented herein.*

SECTION 1: DIABETES MELLITUS

Pearl 1: Differentiating Type 1 Vs. Type 2 Diabetes

Case Scenario:

A 25-year-old man presents with polyuria, polydipsia, weight loss, and fatigue over two weeks. Random plasma glucose is 320 mg/dL. He reports no family history of diabetes. Ketones are detected in the urine.

Key Points and Algorithms:
- **Type 1 Diabetes:**
    - Autoimmune destruction of β-cells.
    - Onset often <30 years but may occur at any age.
    - Acute symptoms (polyuria, polydipsia, polyphagia, weight loss).
    - **Diagnostic Markers:**
        - Positive autoantibodies: GAD65, ICA, ZnT8.
        - Low or undetectable C-peptide.
        - Presence of ketosis.
- **Type 2 Diabetes:**
    - Insulin resistance and relative insulin deficiency.
    - Common in adults, often associated with obesity.
    - Gradual onset, asymptomatic early.

- **Diagnostic Markers:**
  - Elevated C-peptide.
  - No autoantibodies.
  - Often associated with metabolic syndrome.

Tips and Pitfalls:
- Don't overlook Type 1 diabetes in adults—**latent autoimmune diabetes in adults (LADA)** mimics Type 2 diabetes initially.
- Early recognition of ketosis in patients presenting with weight loss and hyperglycemia is crucial to prevent DKA.

MCQ:
A 45-year-old obese patient presents with hyperglycemia but no ketosis. Which test differentiates Type 1 from Type 2 diabetes?
- A) Fasting glucose
- B) HbA1c
- C) C-peptide and GAD65 antibody test
- D) Oral glucose tolerance test
  Answer: C

Clinical Guidelines:
Refer to ADA Standards of Care (2024): Screening for autoantibodies in atypical diabetes presentations.

Pearl 2: Management Of Diabetic Ketoacidosis (Dka)

Case Scenario:

A 19-year-old with Type 1 diabetes presents with nausea, vomiting, abdominal pain, and confusion. Blood glucose: 450 mg/dL, pH: 7.2, bicarbonate: 12 mmol/L, urine ketones: positive.

Key Points and Algorithms:
- **Pathophysiology:** Absolute insulin deficiency → Lipolysis → Ketogenesis → Metabolic acidosis.
- **Management Steps:**
    1. **Fluid Resuscitation:** Start with 0.9% saline. Correct deficits over 24–48 hours.
    2. **Insulin Therapy:** IV regular insulin at 0.1 units/kg/hour.
    3. **Potassium Replacement:** Monitor K+ levels. Replace if <5.3 mmol/L.
    4. **Bicarbonate:** Consider only if pH <6.9.
    5. **Address Precipitating Factors:** Infection, missed insulin doses, etc.

Tips and Pitfalls:
- Monitor potassium closely—**insulin drives K+ intracellularly, risking hypokalemia.**
- Transition to subcutaneous insulin once DKA resolves, with basal insulin overlap to prevent rebound hyperglycemia.

MCQ:
A patient in DKA has a serum potassium of 3.0 mmol/L. What should be the immediate step?
- A) Start IV insulin infusion.
- B) Administer potassium before starting insulin.
- C) Begin bicarbonate therapy.

- D) Give IV fluids only.

  Answer: B

Clinical Guidelines:

Follow ADA guidelines for fluid replacement and insulin protocols in DKA.

Pearl 3: Hypoglycemia In Diabetes

Case Scenario:
A 60-year-old man with Type 2 diabetes on insulin glargine and glimepiride presents with confusion and sweating. Blood glucose: 50 mg/dL.

Key Points and Algorithms:
- **Causes:**
  - Excess insulin or sulfonylurea use.
  - Missed meals or increased physical activity.
  - Alcohol consumption without food.
- **Management:**
  1. Conscious patients: Administer 15–20 g of glucose orally.
  2. Unconscious patients: IV dextrose 25–50 mL of D50% or glucagon 1 mg IM.
  3. Identify and address the cause.

Tips and Pitfalls:
- Avoid overtreatment—**check glucose 15 minutes after treatment and retreat only if necessary.**
- Counsel on meal timing and carb counting to prevent recurrence.

MCQ:
Which of the following is the most appropriate management for an unconscious patient with hypoglycemia?
- A) Oral glucose tablet.

- B) 25–50 mL of D50% IV.
- C) 15 g of glucose.
- D) IV saline.

Answer: B

Clinical Guidelines:

Individualize glycemic targets to avoid hypoglycemia, especially in elderly patients.

Pearl 4: Insulin Regimens And Adjustment

Case Scenario:

A 45-year-old woman with Type 2 diabetes has an HbA1c of 9.2% despite oral agents. She is started on basal-bolus insulin.

Key Points and Algorithms:
- **Insulin Types:**
    - Basal: Long-acting (glargine, detemir).
    - Bolus: Rapid-acting (lispro, aspart).
- **Starting Doses:**
    - Basal insulin: 10 units or 0.1–0.2 units/kg/day.
    - Bolus insulin: 4–6 units before meals or 10% of basal dose per meal.
- **Adjustment:**
    - Adjust based on glucose patterns: **2–4 units every 3 days** or per sliding scale.

Tips and Pitfalls:
- Always teach patients how to recognize and treat hypoglycemia before initiating insulin.

- Ensure proper injection technique to avoid lipohypertrophy.

MCQ:

A patient on basal insulin has fasting glucose levels consistently above 130 mg/dL. What adjustment is appropriate?
- A) Add bolus insulin before breakfast.
- B) Increase basal insulin by 2–4 units.
- C) Decrease basal insulin.
- D) Add a GLP-1 receptor agonist.

Answer: B

Clinical Guidelines:

ADA recommends basal-bolus therapy in uncontrolled Type 2 diabetes after oral agents fail.

Pearl 5: Managing Diabetes In Special Populations

Elderly:
- Prioritize hypoglycemia prevention; relax HbA1c targets (7.5–8%).

Pregnancy:
- Insulin is the preferred treatment. Maintain fasting glucose <95 mg/dL and postprandial <140 mg/dL.

Pediatric:
- Emphasize parental education. Screen for psychosocial issues.

Pearl 6: Advances In Diabetes Technology

- **CGM:** Continuous monitoring reduces HbA1c and hypoglycemia risk.
- **Insulin Pumps:** Ideal for patients with erratic glucose levels or frequent hypoglycemia.

SECTION 2: THYROID DISORDERS

Pearl 7: Approach To Thyroid Nodules

Case Scenario:

A 45-year-old woman presents with an incidentally discovered thyroid nodule on a routine ultrasound. She has no symptoms, and her thyroid function tests are normal.

Key Points and Algorithms:
- **Evaluation Steps:**
    1. **History and Physical Examination:**
        - Risk factors: family history of thyroid cancer, radiation exposure, rapid growth.
        - Symptoms: dysphagia, voice changes.
    2. **Thyroid Function Tests (TFTs):**
        - Measure TSH. Low TSH suggests a hyperfunctioning nodule.
    3. **Thyroid Ultrasound:**
        - Assess size, echogenicity, margins, microcalcifications, and vascularity.
    4. **TIRADS Classification (Thyroid Imaging Reporting and Data System):**
        - Score based on ultrasound features.
        - **TIRADS 1–2:** Benign, no biopsy.
        - **TIRADS 3–5:** Biopsy if ≥1 cm.

Tips and Pitfalls:
- Avoid unnecessary biopsies for small, low-risk nodules (<1 cm, TIRADS 2–3).
- Always correlate ultrasound findings with clinical risk factors.

MCQ:
A patient has a thyroid nodule measuring 2 cm with irregular margins and microcalcifications. TIRADS score is 5. What is the next step?
- A) Repeat ultrasound in 6 months.
- B) Fine-needle aspiration biopsy (FNAB).
- C) Thyroidectomy.
- D) Monitor clinically.
  Answer: B

Clinical Guidelines:
Follow ATA (American Thyroid Association) guidelines for risk stratification and biopsy indications.

Pearl 8: Hyperthyroidism Vs. Thyrotoxicosis

Case Scenario:
A 30-year-old woman presents with palpitations, weight loss, and heat intolerance. TFTs reveal low TSH and elevated free T4.

Key Points and Algorithms:
- Definitions:
  - **Hyperthyroidism:** Overproduction of thyroid hormone (e.g., Graves' disease, toxic nodules).

- **Thyrotoxicosis:** Elevated thyroid hormone levels from any cause (e.g., thyroiditis, exogenous thyroid hormone).
- **Differentiating Causes:**
  - **Graves' disease:** Diffuse goiter, ophthalmopathy, positive TSH receptor antibodies.
  - **Toxic nodule/multinodular goiter:** Hot nodules on radioactive iodine uptake (RAIU).
  - **Thyroiditis:** Low uptake on RAIU due to hormone release from gland destruction.

Management:
1. **Graves' disease:**
   - Beta-blockers for symptom relief.
   - Antithyroid drugs (methimazole or PTU).
   - Radioactive iodine or surgery for definitive treatment.
2. **Toxic nodules:**
   - RAI or surgery.
3. **Thyroiditis:**
   - Symptomatic management with beta-blockers.

Tips and Pitfalls:
- PTU is preferred during the first trimester of pregnancy for Graves' disease.
- Avoid RAI in patients with active ophthalmopathy unless pretreated with steroids.

MCQ:
A 35-year-old patient with thyrotoxicosis has high RAI uptake diffusely. What is the likely diagnosis?

- A) Thyroiditis
- B) Graves' disease
- C) Toxic multinodular goiter
- D) Exogenous thyroid hormone use

Answer: B

Clinical Guidelines:

Use the latest ATA and Endocrine Society guidelines for hyperthyroidism management.

Pearl 9: Hypothyroidism Management

Case Scenario:

A 50-year-old woman with a history of Hashimoto's thyroiditis presents with fatigue, weight gain, and cold intolerance. TSH is elevated, and free T4 is low.

Key Points and Algorithms:

- **Levothyroxine Dosing:**
  - Starting dose: 1.6 mcg/kg/day in young, healthy adults.
  - Start with 12.5–25 mcg/day in elderly or cardiac patients.
  - Adjust every 4–6 weeks based on TSH.
- **Timing of Administration:**
  - Take on an empty stomach, 30–60 minutes before breakfast.
  - Avoid calcium, iron, or antacids for 4 hours.

Tips and Pitfalls:

- Inadequate response may indicate poor adherence,

malabsorption, or drug interactions (e.g., PPI, estrogen).
- Avoid overtreatment, particularly in elderly patients, to prevent osteoporosis or atrial fibrillation.

MCQ:

A patient is taking levothyroxine 100 mcg but remains symptomatic with TSH of 6.5 mIU/L. What is the next step?
- A) Increase dose by 25 mcg.
- B) Add liothyronine.
- C) Test for adrenal insufficiency.
- D) Check for interfering medications.
  Answer: D

Clinical Guidelines:

Refer to ATA guidelines for hypothyroidism management.

Pearl 10: Thyroid Disorders In Pregnancy

Case Scenario:

A 28-year-old pregnant woman at 8 weeks' gestation is diagnosed with hypothyroidism (TSH 5.5 mIU/L, low free T4).

Key Points and Algorithms:
- **Hypothyroidism:**
    - Target TSH <2.5 mIU/L in the first trimester.
    - Increase levothyroxine dose by 30–50% upon confirmation of pregnancy.
- **Hyperthyroidism:**
    - Treat with PTU in the first trimester, switch to methimazole after 12 weeks.
    - Monitor fetal growth and maternal TFTs regularly.

Impact:
- Hypothyroidism: Risk of miscarriage, preeclampsia, and impaired fetal development.
- Hyperthyroidism: Risk of low birth weight, preterm labor, and thyrotoxic crisis.

Tips and Pitfalls:
- Avoid RAI therapy in pregnancy.
- Maintain close coordination between obstetrician and endocrinologist.

MCQ:

Which medication is preferred for hyperthyroidism in the first trimester of pregnancy?

- A) Methimazole
- B) PTU
- C) Levothyroxine
- D) Beta-blockers

Answer: B

Clinical Guidelines:
Follow ATA recommendations for thyroid dysfunction in pregnancy.

Pearl 11: Thyroid Cancer Essentials

Key Points:
- **Papillary Thyroid Cancer (PTC):**
    - Most common, excellent prognosis.
    - Spread: Lymphatic.
    - Treatment: Surgery ± radioactive iodine (RAI).
- **Follicular Thyroid Cancer (FTC):**
    - Spread: Hematogenous (bones, lungs).
    - Treatment: Surgery ± RAI.
- **Medullary Thyroid Cancer (MTC):**
    - Arises from parafollicular C-cells.
    - Associated with MEN2 syndromes.
    - Treatment: Surgery.

Pearl 12: Subclinical Thyroid Disease

Key Points:
- **Subclinical Hypothyroidism:**
    - Elevated TSH, normal free T4.

- Treat if TSH >10 mIU/L, or in symptomatic patients with TSH >7 mIU/L.
- **Subclinical Hyperthyroidism:**
  - Suppressed TSH, normal free T4.
  - Treat if TSH <0.1 mIU/L in elderly or those with cardiac risk.

Clinical Guidelines:

ATA recommends individualized treatment decisions based on age, symptoms, and comorbidities.

SECTION 3: ADRENAL DISORDERS

Pearl 13: Diagnosing Adrenal Insufficiency

Case Scenario:

A 35-year-old man presents with fatigue, weight loss, and hyperpigmentation of his skin. His blood pressure is 90/60 mmHg, and laboratory tests show hyponatremia and hyperkalemia.

Key Points and Algorithms:

- **Types of Adrenal Insufficiency:**
    - **Primary (Addison's Disease):** Adrenal gland dysfunction.
        - Symptoms: Hyperpigmentation, hypotension, fatigue, salt cravings.
        - Labs: Hyponatremia, hyperkalemia, low cortisol, high ACTH.
    - **Secondary:** Pituitary or hypothalamic dysfunction.
        - Symptoms: Similar but no hyperpigmentation.
        - Labs: Low cortisol, low ACTH, normal electrolytes.
- **Diagnostic Workup:**
    1. **Morning Serum Cortisol:** <3 mcg/dL confirms insufficiency; >15 mcg/dL excludes it.

2. **ACTH Stimulation Test:**
   - Administer synthetic ACTH (cosyntropin).
   - Cortisol <18 mcg/dL after stimulation suggests adrenal insufficiency.
3. **Plasma ACTH Levels:**
   - High ACTH: Primary adrenal insufficiency.
   - Low ACTH: Secondary or tertiary adrenal insufficiency.

Tips and Pitfalls:

- Avoid interpreting random cortisol levels without considering timing and context.
- In acute illness, a single low cortisol (<10 mcg/dL) supports the diagnosis of adrenal crisis.

MCQ:

A patient with suspected adrenal insufficiency has morning cortisol of 2 mcg/dL and elevated ACTH. What is the likely diagnosis?

- A) Primary adrenal insufficiency
- B) Secondary adrenal insufficiency
- C) Tertiary adrenal insufficiency
- D) Adrenal hyperplasia

Answer: A

Clinical Guidelines:

Follow Endocrine Society guidelines for diagnosis and treatment of adrenal insufficiency.

Pearl 14: Cushing's Syndrome

Case Scenario:
A 50-year-old woman presents with central obesity, a round face, purple striae, and proximal muscle weakness. Laboratory tests show hyperglycemia and hypertension.

Key Points and Algorithms:
- **Causes of Cushing's Syndrome:**
    1. **ACTH-Dependent:** Pituitary adenoma (Cushing's disease), ectopic ACTH.
    2. **ACTH-Independent:** Adrenal adenoma, exogenous glucocorticoids.
- **Diagnostic Tests:**
    1. **Screening Tests:**
        - **1 mg Overnight Dexamethasone Suppression Test:**
            - Cortisol >5 mcg/dL confirms hypercortisolism.
        - **24-Hour Urine Free Cortisol:** Elevated in Cushing's syndrome.
        - **Late-Night Salivary Cortisol:** Elevated in Cushing's syndrome.
    2. **Confirmatory Tests:**
        - Plasma ACTH to differentiate ACTH-dependent vs. independent causes.
    3. **Imaging:**
        - Pituitary MRI, adrenal CT, or whole-

body scan for ectopic ACTH.
- **Management:**
  - **Pituitary Adenoma:** Transsphenoidal surgery.
  - **Adrenal Tumor:** Adrenalectomy.
  - **Ectopic ACTH:** Treat underlying malignancy.
  - **Medical Therapy:** Ketoconazole, metyrapone, or mitotane for unresectable cases.

Tips and Pitfalls:
- Avoid screening during acute illness or stress, which can transiently elevate cortisol.
- Differentiate pseudo-Cushing's (e.g., obesity, depression) with additional testing.

MCQ:
Which test is most appropriate for screening Cushing's syndrome?
- A) Morning serum cortisol
- B) Late-night salivary cortisol
- C) Plasma ACTH
- D) Serum aldosterone

Answer: B

Clinical Guidelines:
Refer to Endocrine Society guidelines for diagnosis and management.

Pearl 15: Pheochromocytoma And Paragangliomas

Case Scenario:

A 40-year-old woman presents with episodic headaches, palpitations, and sweating. Her blood pressure is 180/110 mmHg during an episode.

Key Points and Algorithms:
- **Classic Triad:** Headache, palpitations, sweating (present in 90% of cases).
- **Diagnostic Tests:**
    1. **Plasma Free Metanephrines:** Highly sensitive for pheochromocytoma.
    2. **24-Hour Urine Metanephrines and Catecholamines:** To confirm diagnosis.
    3. **Imaging:** CT or MRI of adrenal glands; whole-body scan for extra-adrenal paragangliomas.
- **Preoperative Management:**
    1. **Alpha-Blockade:** Phenoxybenzamine (start 10–14 days before surgery).
    2. **Beta-Blockade:** Add only after adequate alpha-blockade to control tachycardia.
    3. **Hydration:** Liberal fluid intake to prevent hypotension postoperatively.
- **Surgical Approach:**
    - Laparoscopic adrenalectomy is preferred.

Tips and Pitfalls:
- Always initiate alpha-blockade before beta-blockade to avoid unopposed alpha stimulation and hypertensive crisis.
- Screen for genetic syndromes (e.g., MEN2, VHL) in young or bilateral cases.

MCQ:

A patient with pheochromocytoma is scheduled for surgery. What is the first step in preoperative preparation?
- A) Administer beta-blockers.
- B) Administer alpha-blockers.
- C) Perform adrenal CT scan.
- D) Start antihypertensive therapy with ACE inhibitors.

Answer: B

Clinical Guidelines:
Follow international consensus guidelines for pheochromocytoma and paragangliomas.

Section 4: Pituitary Disorders

Pearl 16: Recognizing Pituitary Tumors

Case Scenario:
A 45-year-old woman presents with headaches, amenorrhea, and decreased libido. Visual field testing reveals bitemporal hemianopia.

Key Points and Algorithms:
- **Types of Pituitary Tumors:**
    1. **Functioning Tumors:** Secrete hormones (e.g., prolactinoma, growth hormone-secreting tumor).
    2. **Non-Functioning Tumors:** Do not secrete active hormones but cause symptoms through mass effect.
- **Common Presentations:**
    - **Hormonal Excess Symptoms:**
        - **Prolactinoma:** Galactorrhea,

amenorrhea, infertility in women; decreased libido and erectile dysfunction in men.
- **Acromegaly:** Enlarged hands/feet, coarsened facial features, joint pain.
- **Cushing's Disease:** Symptoms of hypercortisolism (Pearl 14).

○ **Mass Effect Symptoms:**
- Headaches, visual field defects (bitemporal hemianopia), hypopituitarism.

- **Diagnostic Workup:**
  1. **Hormonal Tests:**
     - Prolactin, IGF-1, ACTH, cortisol, TSH, free T4, LH/FSH, testosterone/estradiol.
  2. **Imaging:**
     - **MRI with Gadolinium Contrast:** Gold standard for pituitary imaging.

- **Management:**
  ○ **Prolactinoma:** Dopamine agonists (e.g., cabergoline).
  ○ **Other Tumors:** Surgical resection (transsphenoidal approach) for symptomatic or nonresponsive tumors.
  ○ **Radiotherapy or Medical Therapy:** For recurrent or inoperable cases.

Tips and Pitfalls:
- Always exclude macroprolactin interference in

prolactin assays.
- Be cautious about pituitary apoplexy presenting with sudden headache and hormonal crisis.

MCQ:

A patient with a pituitary tumor has bitemporal hemianopia and elevated prolactin levels. What is the most likely diagnosis?
- A) Non-functioning adenoma
- B) Craniopharyngioma
- C) Prolactinoma
- D) Pituitary apoplexy

Answer: C

Clinical Guidelines:

Refer to the Pituitary Society guidelines for evaluation and treatment of pituitary tumors.

Pearl 17: Diabetes Insipidus And Siadh

Case Scenario:

A 50-year-old man presents with excessive thirst and polyuria. Urine output is 6 liters/day, and lab results show low urine osmolality with high serum sodium.

Key Points and Algorithms:
- **Diabetes Insipidus (DI):**
  - **Definition:** Impaired water reabsorption due to insufficient ADH (central DI) or renal resistance to ADH (nephrogenic DI).
  - **Symptoms:** Polyuria, polydipsia, nocturia, dehydration.

- **Diagnostic Tests:**
    1. **Serum and Urine Osmolality:**
        - High serum osmolality, low urine osmolality.
    2. **Water Deprivation Test:**
        - In DI, urine osmolality remains low despite dehydration.
    3. **Response to Desmopressin:**
        - Improvement: Central DI.
        - No improvement: Nephrogenic DI.

- **Syndrome of Inappropriate Antidiuretic Hormone Secretion (SIADH):**
    - **Definition:** Excessive ADH secretion leading to water retention and hyponatremia.
    - **Symptoms:** Nausea, confusion, seizures in severe cases.
    - **Diagnostic Tests:**
        1. **Serum and Urine Osmolality:**
            - Low serum osmolality, high urine osmolality, low serum sodium.
        2. **Exclusion of Other Causes:** Hypothyroidism, adrenal insufficiency.

- **Management:**
    - **DI:**
        - **Central DI:** Desmopressin (DDAVP).
        - **Nephrogenic DI:** Thiazide diuretics, low-sodium diet, manage underlying cause.

- **SIADH:**
  - Fluid restriction, salt tablets, loop diuretics.
  - Severe cases: Hypertonic saline with close monitoring.

Tips and Pitfalls:
- Do not start hypertonic saline in SIADH without calculating the sodium correction rate (avoid central pontine myelinolysis).
- Polyuria in DI can mimic uncontrolled diabetes mellitus—always check urine glucose.

MCQ:

Which of the following distinguishes central diabetes insipidus from nephrogenic diabetes insipidus?
- A) Response to water deprivation test
- B) Serum osmolality
- C) Response to desmopressin
- D) Presence of hyponatremia
  Answer: C

Clinical Guidelines:

Follow the latest Endocrine Society guidelines on the diagnosis and treatment of fluid balance disorders.

SECTION 5: CALCIUM AND BONE DISORDERS

Pearl 18: Hypercalcemia And Primary Hyperparathyroidism

Case Scenario:
A 65-year-old woman presents with fatigue, muscle weakness, and frequent urination. Blood tests reveal serum calcium of 11.8 mg/dL, elevated parathyroid hormone (PTH), and low phosphate levels.

Key Points and Algorithms:
- **Common Causes of Hypercalcemia:**
    1. **Primary Hyperparathyroidism (PHPT):**
        - Elevated PTH, hypercalcemia, hypophosphatemia.
        - Common in postmenopausal women.
    2. **Malignancy:**
        - Associated with PTH-related protein (PTHrP) or bone metastases.
    3. **Other Causes:** Vitamin D toxicity, granulomatous diseases, medications (e.g., thiazides).
- **Clinical Presentation:**
    ◦ "Stones, bones, abdominal groans, and psychic moans": Kidney stones, bone pain, GI

symptoms, neuropsychiatric changes.
- **Diagnostic Workup:**
  - **Laboratory Tests:** Serum calcium, ionized calcium, PTH, 25-hydroxyvitamin D, phosphate.
  - **Imaging:**
    - Ultrasound or Sestamibi scan for parathyroid adenoma.
- **Management of Hypercalcemia:**
  - **Mild (Ca <12 mg/dL):** Encourage hydration; monitor.
  - **Moderate to Severe (>14 mg/dL):**
    1. **Acute Management:**
       - IV fluids, loop diuretics (e.g., furosemide).
       - Bisphosphonates (e.g., zoledronic acid).
       - Calcitonin for rapid calcium reduction.
    2. **Long-Term Management for PHPT:**
       - Surgical removal of parathyroid adenoma.
       - Cinacalcet if surgery is contraindicated.

Tips and Pitfalls:
- Always correct calcium for albumin levels in lab results.
- Rule out malignancy promptly in cases of severe hypercalcemia.

MCQ:
A patient with hypercalcemia, elevated PTH, and low phosphate likely

has:

- A) Malignancy-associated hypercalcemia
- B) Primary hyperparathyroidism
- C) Vitamin D toxicity
- D) Chronic kidney disease

  Answer: B

Clinical Guidelines:

Follow the American Association of Clinical Endocrinologists (AACE) guidelines for hyperparathyroidism evaluation and treatment.

Pearl 19: Osteoporosis Management

Case Scenario:
A 70-year-old postmenopausal woman with a history of a vertebral compression fracture has a T-score of -2.8 on dual-energy X-ray absorptiometry (DXA).

Key Points and Algorithms:
- **Risk Factors:**
    - Aging, menopause, glucocorticoid use, smoking, alcohol, family history of fractures.
- **Diagnosis:**
    - **DXA Scan:** T-score ≤ -2.5 indicates osteoporosis.
    - **FRAX Tool:** Estimates 10-year fracture risk to guide treatment decisions.
- **Pharmacologic Options:**
    1. **Antiresorptive Agents:**
        - Bisphosphonates (e.g., alendronate, zoledronic acid).
        - Denosumab: Effective for high-risk patients.
    2. **Anabolic Agents:**
        - Teriparatide or abaloparatide for severe cases.
    3. **Others:** Raloxifene (for postmenopausal women); hormone replacement therapy in select cases.
- **Lifestyle Modifications:**
    - Calcium (1200 mg/day) and Vitamin D (800 IU/day) supplementation.

- Weight-bearing exercise, fall prevention strategies.
- **Monitoring:**
  - Repeat DXA every 1-2 years for treatment response.

Tips and Pitfalls:
- Avoid oversupplementation with calcium, which can increase cardiovascular risk.
- Screen men over 70 and postmenopausal women for osteoporosis risk.

MCQ:
Which of the following medications is anabolic and stimulates new bone formation in osteoporosis?
- A) Alendronate
- B) Teriparatide
- C) Denosumab
- D) Raloxifene

Answer: B

Clinical Guidelines:
Refer to the National Osteoporosis Foundation (NOF) guidelines for prevention and treatment.

Pearl 20: Hypocalcemia

Case Scenario:
A 55-year-old man presents with muscle cramps, tingling around the mouth, and a positive Chvostek's sign. Serum calcium is 7.2 mg/dL, with low PTH levels.

Key Points and Algorithms:
- **Causes of Hypocalcemia:**
    - **Low PTH:** Hypoparathyroidism (post-surgical, autoimmune).
    - **High PTH:** Vitamin D deficiency, chronic kidney disease, pseudohypoparathyroidism.
- **Clinical Presentation:**
    - Neuromuscular irritability: Tetany, carpopedal spasms, seizures.
    - Prolonged QT interval on ECG.
- **Diagnostic Workup:**
    - Serum calcium (corrected for albumin), ionized calcium, PTH, magnesium, 25-hydroxyvitamin D.
- **Management:**
    - **Acute Symptomatic Hypocalcemia:**
        1. IV calcium gluconate.
        2. Address underlying causes (e.g., magnesium deficiency).
    - **Chronic Hypocalcemia:**
        - Oral calcium supplements.
        - Vitamin D (calcitriol) for hypoparathyroidism.

Tips and Pitfalls:
- Always correct magnesium deficiency before treating hypocalcemia.
- In chronic hypocalcemia, avoid overtreatment to prevent hypercalciuria and kidney stones.

MCQ:

A patient with hypocalcemia, low PTH, and a history of neck surgery most likely has:
- A) Vitamin D deficiency
- B) Chronic kidney disease
- C) Primary hypoparathyroidism
- D) Pseudohypoparathyroidism

Answer: C

Clinical Guidelines:

Use the Endocrine Society's guidelines on hypocalcemia management for tailored treatment plans.

SECTION 6: MISCELLANEOUS HORMONAL DISORDERS

Pearl 21: Polycystic Ovary Syndrome (Pcos)

Case Scenario:

A 25-year-old woman presents with irregular periods, hirsutism, and difficulty losing weight. An ultrasound shows multiple ovarian follicles, and lab results reveal elevated total testosterone and normal thyroid and prolactin levels.

Key Points and Algorithms:

- **Diagnostic Criteria (Rotterdam Criteria, 2 out of 3 required):**
    1. Oligo- or anovulation (irregular menstrual cycles).
    2. Hyperandrogenism (clinical or biochemical).
    3. Polycystic ovarian morphology on ultrasound (>12 follicles per ovary or ovarian volume >10 mL).
- **Pathophysiology:**
    - Insulin resistance and hyperinsulinemia contribute to hyperandrogenism.
- **Management:**
    1. **Lifestyle Modifications:**
        - Weight loss and exercise to improve insulin sensitivity.
    2. **Medical Therapy:**

- **For Menstrual Irregularity:**
  - Combined oral contraceptives (COCs) to regulate cycles and lower androgen levels.
- **For Hyperandrogenism:**
  - Antiandrogens (e.g., spironolactone) after contraception is ensured.
- **For Insulin Resistance:**
  - Metformin to improve insulin sensitivity and ovulatory function.
- **For Infertility:**
  - Letrozole as the first-line ovulation induction agent.

Tips and Pitfalls:
- Always rule out other causes of hyperandrogenism, such as congenital adrenal hyperplasia or androgen-secreting tumors.
- Monitor for metabolic complications like diabetes and dyslipidemia.

MCQ:
Which medication is first-line for ovulation induction in PCOS patients seeking pregnancy?
- A) Clomiphene citrate
- B) Letrozole
- C) Metformin
- D) Spironolactone

Answer: B

Clinical Guidelines:
Follow the Endocrine Society's Clinical Practice Guideline for PCOS.

Pearl 22: Hypogonadism In Males And Females

Case Scenario:
A 45-year-old man complains of fatigue, decreased libido, and muscle weakness. Labs show low total testosterone and normal luteinizing hormone (LH) and follicle-stimulating hormone (FSH) levels.

Key Points and Algorithms:
- **Types of Hypogonadism:**
    1. **Primary (Hypergonadotropic):** Testicular or ovarian failure (elevated LH/FSH).
    2. **Secondary (Hypogonadotropic):** Pituitary or hypothalamic dysfunction (low LH/FSH).
- **Diagnosis:**
    - **Males:** Morning total testosterone levels (repeat abnormal tests).
    - **Females:** Low estradiol with menopausal symptoms in premenopausal women.
    - Assess LH, FSH, prolactin, iron studies (hemochromatosis), and MRI for secondary causes.
- **Management:**
    1. **Testosterone Replacement Therapy (TRT) in Men:**
        - Indicated for symptomatic hypogonadism with low testosterone.
        - Routes: Transdermal gel, intramuscular injections, or patches.
        - Monitor hematocrit, PSA, and lipid

profile.
2. **Estrogen/Progesterone Therapy in Women:**
   - Premature ovarian insufficiency or menopausal symptoms.
   - Use lowest effective dose and reassess regularly.

Tips and Pitfalls:
- Avoid TRT in men with prostate cancer or high hematocrit.
- In women, ensure contraindications like active thromboembolic disease are ruled out before starting hormone therapy.

MCQ:
Which of the following is a contraindication for testosterone replacement therapy in men?
- A) Sleep apnea
- B) History of prostate cancer
- C) Dyslipidemia
- D) Osteoporosis

Answer: B

Clinical Guidelines:
Refer to the American Urological Association (AUA) guidelines for male hypogonadism and the North American Menopause Society (NAMS) guidelines for hormone therapy in women.

Pearl 23: Disorders Of Puberty

Case Scenario:
A 7-year-old girl presents with early breast development and pubic hair. Bone age is advanced compared to chronological age.

Key Points and Algorithms:
- **Normal Puberty:**
    - Begins between 8-13 years in girls, 9-14 years in boys.
- **Precocious Puberty:**
    - **Central (Gonadotropin-Dependent):** Early activation of the hypothalamic-pituitary-gonadal axis (e.g., idiopathic, CNS tumors).
    - **Peripheral (Gonadotropin-Independent):** Excess sex steroid production (e.g., adrenal tumors, McCune-Albright syndrome).
- **Delayed Puberty:**
    - No signs of puberty by age 13 in girls or 14 in boys.
    - **Causes:** Constitutional delay, hypogonadism, chronic illness, malnutrition.
- **Diagnostic Workup:**
    - LH, FSH, estradiol/testosterone, bone age assessment.
    - MRI for central causes if LH/FSH is elevated in precocious puberty.
- **Management:**
    1. **Precocious Puberty:**
        - GnRH agonists for central precocious puberty.
        - Treat underlying cause in peripheral cases.
    2. **Delayed Puberty:**
        - Testosterone or estrogen therapy for hypogonadism.

- Monitor growth and sexual development.

Tips and Pitfalls:

- In precocious puberty, differentiate benign variants (e.g., premature thelarche) from pathological causes.
- In delayed puberty, rule out Turner syndrome in girls and Klinefelter syndrome in boys.

MCQ:

A child with precocious puberty and low LH levels even after GnRH stimulation likely has:

- A) Central precocious puberty
- B) Peripheral precocious puberty
- C) Constitutional delay of puberty
- D) Hypogonadotropic hypogonadism
  Answer: B

Clinical Guidelines:

Use the Pediatric Endocrine Society's guidelines for the evaluation and management of precocious and delayed puberty.

50 QUESTIONS ON ENDOCRINOLOGY

Question 1:

Q: *A 45-year-old man presents with polyuria, polydipsia, and weight loss. A random plasma glucose is 230 mg/dL, and HbA1c is 8.5%. What is the diagnosis?*

- A) Type 1 Diabetes
- B) Type 2 Diabetes
- C) Impaired Glucose Tolerance
- D) Gestational Diabetes

Answer:
B) Type 2 Diabetes

Explanation:

- **Diagnostic Criteria for Diabetes (American Diabetes Association):**
    1. Fasting Plasma Glucose (FPG) ≥126 mg/dL.
    2. 2-hour OGTT ≥200 mg/dL.
    3. Random Plasma Glucose ≥200 mg/dL with symptoms.
    4. HbA1c ≥6.5%.
- This patient meets the criteria with an HbA1c of 8.5% and a random glucose of 230 mg/dL.

Pitfalls:

- Missing the diagnosis if a fasting glucose alone is used (some cases only manifest with postprandial

hyperglycemia).
- Overlooking potential underlying Type 1 diabetes in adults with ketosis or rapid weight loss.

Pearls:

- Always confirm the diagnosis with a repeat test unless symptoms and glucose >200 mg/dL are definitive.
- Screen for complications at the time of diagnosis (e.g., retinopathy, nephropathy).

Question 2:

Q: *A patient has TSH = 0.2 µIU/mL (low) and free T4 = 2.8 ng/dL (high). What is the most likely diagnosis?*
- A) Primary Hypothyroidism
- B) Graves' Disease
- C) Subclinical Hyperthyroidism
- D) Thyroiditis

Answer:
B) Graves' Disease

Explanation:
- **Graves' Disease** is an autoimmune condition characterized by thyroid-stimulating antibodies causing hyperthyroidism.
- Lab findings: Low TSH, elevated free T4.
- Clinical findings: Weight loss, palpitations, exophthalmos, and goiter.

Pitfalls:
- Not checking TSH receptor antibody (TRAb) levels to confirm Graves'.
- Assuming all hyperthyroidism cases are Graves'; consider toxic multinodular goiter or thyroiditis.

Pearls:
- Radioactive iodine uptake scan can differentiate Graves' from thyroiditis.
- Beta-blockers provide symptom relief while definitive therapy (radioiodine, antithyroid drugs) is planned.

Question 3:

Q: *Which of the following tests is most appropriate for diagnosing primary adrenal insufficiency?*

- A) Plasma Renin Activity
- B) Morning Serum Cortisol
- C) ACTH Stimulation Test
- D) Serum Aldosterone

Answer:

C) ACTH Stimulation Test

Explanation:

- In primary adrenal insufficiency, the adrenal glands fail to respond to ACTH stimulation, resulting in low cortisol levels post-stimulation.
- Morning cortisol levels can be misleading in early disease.

Pitfalls:

- Failure to differentiate primary from secondary adrenal insufficiency; in secondary, ACTH is low, and aldosterone is typically preserved.
- Relying solely on serum cortisol without confirmatory ACTH stimulation.

Pearls:

- Check electrolytes; hyperkalemia and hyponatremia are common in primary adrenal insufficiency.
- Initiate glucocorticoid therapy immediately if adrenal crisis is suspected.

Question 4:

Q: *What is the first-line treatment for severe hypercalcemia (>14 mg/dL)?*

- A) Oral Bisphosphonates

- B) IV Hydration with Normal Saline
- C) Calcitonin
- D) Hemodialysis

Answer:
B) IV Hydration with Normal Saline

Explanation:
- Hypercalcemia often leads to dehydration due to polyuria. Hydration corrects volume depletion and promotes calcium excretion.
- Calcitonin and bisphosphonates are second-line therapies.

Pitfalls:
- Ignoring the underlying cause of hypercalcemia (e.g., malignancy, primary hyperparathyroidism).
- Delaying bisphosphonates, which are essential for sustained calcium reduction in malignancy.

Pearls:
- Reassess calcium levels frequently during treatment.
- Address the root cause of hypercalcemia alongside symptomatic management.

Question 5:

Q: *A 32-year-old woman presents with amenorrhea, galactorrhea, and headaches. What is the first test you should order?*
- A) MRI of the Brain
- B) Serum Prolactin Level
- C) LH and FSH
- D) Visual Field Testing

Answer:
B) Serum Prolactin Level

Explanation:

- Symptoms suggest hyperprolactinemia, commonly caused by a prolactinoma. Prolactin measurement is the most appropriate initial test.
- If prolactin is elevated, MRI is indicated to confirm a pituitary lesion.

Pitfalls:

- Not ruling out other causes of hyperprolactinemia, such as medications (e.g., antipsychotics) or hypothyroidism.
- Missing visual field defects in large tumors compressing the optic chiasm.

Pearls:

- Dopamine agonists (e.g., cabergoline) are effective first-line treatments for prolactinomas.
- Surgical intervention is rarely required unless medical therapy fails.

Question 6:

Q: *Which of the following is the first-line pharmacological treatment for irregular menses in PCOS?*

- A) Metformin
- B) Combined Oral Contraceptives (COCs)
- C) Clomiphene Citrate
- D) Spironolactone

Answer:
B) Combined Oral Contraceptives (COCs)
Explanation:

- COCs regulate menstrual cycles, reduce androgen

levels, and protect the endometrium.
- Metformin improves insulin resistance but is not the first choice for cycle regulation.

Pitfalls:
- Using spironolactone without adequate contraception due to teratogenic risks.
- Failing to address lifestyle changes, which are the cornerstone of PCOS management.

Pearls:
- Always assess and address metabolic risks, including diabetes and dyslipidemia.
- Clomiphene is first-line for ovulation induction in women desiring pregnancy.

Question 7:

Q: *A 29-year-old woman presents with fatigue, dry skin, and weight gain. Her TSH is 8 µIU/mL, and free T4 is within normal limits. What is the most likely diagnosis?*
- A) Subclinical Hypothyroidism
- B) Primary Hypothyroidism
- C) Euthyroid Sick Syndrome
- D) Central Hypothyroidism

Answer:
A) Subclinical Hypothyroidism

Explanation:
- Subclinical hypothyroidism is characterized by elevated TSH with normal free T4 levels.
- Patients are often asymptomatic, but mild symptoms may appear.

Pitfalls:

- Starting levothyroxine therapy without a clear indication (e.g., TSH >10 or pregnancy).
- Missing secondary causes, such as thyroiditis or iodine deficiency.

Pearls:

- Treat if TSH >10 µIU/mL, or if symptomatic with TSH between 4.5–10 µIU/mL.
- Monitor TSH periodically in asymptomatic cases.

Question 8:

Q: *Which of the following is a contraindication to metformin therapy?*

- A) Chronic Kidney Disease with eGFR <30 mL/min/1.73 m²
- B) Mild Hepatic Impairment
- C) History of PCOS
- D) Obesity

Answer:

A) Chronic Kidney Disease with eGFR <30 mL/min/1.73 m²

Explanation:

- Metformin is contraindicated in advanced CKD due to the risk of lactic acidosis.
- It can be cautiously used if eGFR is >30 but <45 mL/min/1.73 m² with dose adjustment.

Pitfalls:

- Overestimating risks in mild renal impairment and unnecessarily withholding metformin.
- Not considering alternatives like SGLT2 inhibitors in CKD patients.

Pearls:

- Metformin remains the first-line agent for Type 2

diabetes unless contraindicated.
- Ensure renal function monitoring every 3–6 months in borderline cases.

Question 9:

Q: *A 46-year-old woman with hypertension and hypokalemia is found to have a plasma aldosterone-to-renin ratio of 35. What is the most likely diagnosis?*

- A) Primary Hyperaldosteronism
- B) Secondary Hyperaldosteronism
- C) Cushing's Syndrome
- D) Pheochromocytoma

Answer:
A) Primary Hyperaldosteronism

Explanation:
- Elevated aldosterone-to-renin ratio (>20) suggests primary hyperaldosteronism, commonly due to adrenal adenoma or hyperplasia.
- Hypokalemia and resistant hypertension are hallmark features.

Pitfalls:
- Failing to confirm with salt suppression testing.
- Overlooking adrenal vein sampling in cases of bilateral adrenal hyperplasia vs. adenoma.

Pearls:
- Spironolactone is the first-line treatment in bilateral disease.
- Surgery is indicated for unilateral adenomas.

Question 10:

Q: *What is the first-line pharmacologic treatment for postmenopausal osteoporosis?*

- A) Bisphosphonates
- B) Denosumab
- C) Teriparatide
- D) Calcitonin

Answer:

A) Bisphosphonates

Explanation:

- Bisphosphonates (e.g., alendronate) inhibit bone resorption and are first-line in most cases.
- Other agents like denosumab or teriparatide are reserved for high-risk or intolerant patients.

Pitfalls:

- Overlooking contraindications such as esophageal disorders for oral bisphosphonates.
- Neglecting vitamin D and calcium supplementation.

Pearls:

- Monitor bone density every 1–2 years to assess treatment response.
- Ensure drug holidays after long-term use to reduce atypical fracture risks.

Question 11:

Q: *What is the primary mechanism of action of metformin in managing PCOS?*

- A) Decreases Androgen Production
- B) Improves Insulin Sensitivity
- C) Induces Ovulation
- D) Reduces Hirsutism

Answer:
B) Improves Insulin Sensitivity

Explanation:
- Metformin improves insulin resistance, which is central to PCOS pathophysiology. This, in turn, can indirectly improve ovulation and reduce androgen levels.

Pitfalls:
- Using metformin as first-line therapy for ovulation induction; clomiphene is preferred.
- Overestimating metformin's effect on androgen symptoms like hirsutism.

Pearls:
- Lifestyle modification remains the cornerstone of PCOS management.
- Metformin is particularly beneficial in PCOS patients with diabetes or glucose intolerance.

Question 12:

Q: A 45-year-old patient presents with heat intolerance, weight loss, and palpitations. TSH is suppressed, and free T4 is elevated. A thyroid scan shows diffuse increased uptake. What is the most likely diagnosis?
- A) Graves' Disease
- B) Toxic Multinodular Goiter
- C) Thyroiditis
- D) Thyroid Adenoma

Answer:
A) Graves' Disease

Explanation:

- Diffuse increased uptake on a thyroid scan is diagnostic of Graves' disease, an autoimmune condition characterized by hyperthyroidism.
- Common features include exophthalmos and pretibial myxedema.

Pitfalls:
- Confusing toxic multinodular goiter (patchy uptake) with Graves' disease.
- Missing thyroiditis, which typically shows reduced uptake.

Pearls:
- Radioactive iodine therapy is a preferred treatment in non-pregnant adults.
- Beta-blockers are effective for symptom control.

Question 13:

Q: *A 35-year-old woman with galactorrhea and menstrual irregularity has a serum prolactin level of 120 ng/mL. MRI reveals a 5 mm pituitary adenoma. What is the first-line treatment?*

- A) Surgical Resection
- B) Dopamine Agonists
- C) Radiation Therapy
- D) Observation

Answer:
B) Dopamine Agonists
Explanation:
- Dopamine agonists (e.g., cabergoline or bromocriptine) are the first-line treatment for prolactinomas. They normalize prolactin levels and reduce tumor size.

Pitfalls:

- Misdiagnosing physiologic hyperprolactinemia (e.g., pregnancy).
- Delaying treatment in macroadenomas causing visual field defects.

Pearls:
- Surgery is reserved for dopamine agonist-resistant cases.
- Monitor prolactin levels periodically to assess treatment response.

Question 14:

Q: *What is the confirmatory test for primary adrenal insufficiency?*
- A) ACTH Stimulation Test
- B) Serum Aldosterone Measurement
- C) 24-Hour Urine Cortisol
- D) Salivary Cortisol Test

Answer:
A) ACTH Stimulation Test

Explanation:
- The ACTH stimulation test assesses adrenal gland function by measuring cortisol response to synthetic ACTH. A blunted response confirms adrenal insufficiency.

Pitfalls:
- Overreliance on morning cortisol alone, which can be misleading.
- Misinterpreting low cortisol in critically ill patients without adrenal insufficiency.

Pearls:

- Distinguish primary from secondary adrenal insufficiency by measuring ACTH levels.
- Lifelong glucocorticoid replacement therapy is required for primary adrenal insufficiency.

Question 15:

Q: *Which class of diabetes medications provides cardiovascular benefits in patients with Type 2 Diabetes and established atherosclerotic cardiovascular disease?*

- A) SGLT2 Inhibitors
- B) DPP-4 Inhibitors
- C) Sulfonylureas
- D) Alpha-Glucosidase Inhibitors

Answer:
A) SGLT2 Inhibitors
Explanation:

- SGLT2 inhibitors (e.g., empagliflozin, canagliflozin) reduce cardiovascular risk and heart failure hospitalizations in high-risk patients.

Pitfalls:

- Not screening for eGFR as these drugs are contraindicated in severe renal impairment.
- Overlooking their potential to cause euglycemic DKA.

Pearls:

- GLP-1 receptor agonists also provide cardiovascular benefits.
- Monitor for genitourinary infections, a common side effect.

Question 16:

Q: *A 70-year-old woman presents with a history of recurrent fractures. Her DEXA scan reveals a T-score of -3.0. Which of the following is the best treatment to reduce fracture risk?*

- A) Alendronate
- B) Calcitonin
- C) Calcium Supplementation Alone
- D) Teriparatide

Answer:
A) Alendronate
Explanation:
- Bisphosphonates like alendronate are first-line for osteoporosis due to their strong anti-fracture efficacy in spine and hip fractures.

Pitfalls:
- Ignoring vitamin D status, which is essential for bisphosphonate efficacy.
- Overlooking teriparatide for patients with severe osteoporosis or multiple fractures.

Pearls:
- Patients should remain upright for 30 minutes after taking alendronate to prevent esophageal irritation.
- Reevaluate after 3–5 years to consider a drug holiday.

Question 17:

Q: *Which hormone is the best marker for ovarian reserve?*

- A) Anti-Müllerian Hormone (AMH)

- B) Follicle-Stimulating Hormone (FSH)
- C) Estradiol
- D) Progesterone

Answer:
A) Anti-Müllerian Hormone (AMH)

Explanation:
- AMH is a reliable marker for ovarian reserve as it reflects the remaining follicular pool.
- FSH and estradiol levels vary during the menstrual cycle and are less consistent.

Pitfalls:
- Using AMH levels alone to diagnose infertility.
- Misinterpreting low AMH in younger patients who may still have good fertility potential.

Pearls:
- AMH is not affected by the menstrual cycle, making it convenient for testing.
- Combine AMH with antral follicle count for a comprehensive assessment.

Question 18:

Q: *A 42-year-old man presents with enlarged hands, feet, and facial features. MRI reveals a pituitary mass. His IGF-1 levels are markedly elevated. What is the most appropriate initial treatment?*

- A) Surgical Resection of the Pituitary Tumor
- B) Radiation Therapy
- C) Somatostatin Analogs
- D) Dopamine Agonists

Answer:
A) Surgical Resection of the Pituitary Tumor

Explanation:
- The first-line treatment for acromegaly is usually surgical resection of the pituitary adenoma.
- If surgery is not successful or if the patient is not a surgical candidate, somatostatin analogs (e.g., octreotide) are commonly used.

Pitfalls:
- Failing to assess for other causes of elevated IGF-1, such as ectopic sources.
- Misdiagnosing the condition as simply "aging" when there are subtle features like enlarged hands or feet.

Pearls:
- Post-surgical follow-up with IGF-1 levels and MRI is essential.
- If surgery fails, medical therapies (somatostatin analogs, pegvisomant) or radiation therapy should be considered.

Question 19:

Q: *A 39-year-old woman presents with obesity, purple striae, and easy bruising. Her 24-hour urinary cortisol is elevated. What is the next step in confirming the diagnosis?*
- A) Low-Dose Dexamethasone Suppression Test
- B) Serum ACTH Measurement
- C) MRI of the Adrenal Glands
- D) ACTH Stimulation Test

Answer:
B) Serum ACTH Measurement

Explanation:
- After confirming high cortisol levels, measuring serum

ACTH helps differentiate between ACTH-dependent (e.g., Cushing's disease) and ACTH-independent causes (e.g., adrenal adenoma).
- If ACTH is suppressed, it suggests an adrenal cause; if it is elevated, it points to pituitary involvement or ectopic ACTH secretion.

Pitfalls:

- Misinterpreting cortisol levels in patients with critical illness or depression.
- Failing to distinguish between Cushing's disease and ectopic ACTH production, which requires additional imaging.

Pearls:

- Once ACTH-dependent Cushing's syndrome is confirmed, MRI of the pituitary is performed to identify adenomas.
- Use dexamethasone suppression tests for confirming the diagnosis of Cushing's syndrome in doubtful cases.

Question 20:

Q: *A newborn presents with ambiguous genitalia and is diagnosed with congenital adrenal hyperplasia. What is the first-line treatment to correct the hormonal imbalance?*

- A) Hydrocortisone
- B) Fludrocortisone
- C) Spironolactone
- D) Dexamethasone

Answer:

A) Hydrocortisone

Explanation:
- The mainstay of treatment for CAH is hydrocortisone to replace cortisol and suppress excessive ACTH secretion. Fludrocortisone is also often needed for aldosterone replacement if the salt-wasting form is present.

Pitfalls:
- Misdiagnosing CAH in mild cases, especially non-classic forms, which can present later in life.
- Overcorrecting with steroids, which can lead to Cushingoid symptoms.

Pearls:
- Patients with CAH require lifelong corticosteroid therapy, with regular adjustments to doses, especially during times of illness or stress.
- Genetic counseling should be offered to families with CAH.

Question 21:

Q: A 25-year-old male with anosmia (loss of sense of smell) presents with delayed puberty. What is the most likely diagnosis?
- A) Klinefelter Syndrome
- B) Kallmann Syndrome
- C) Prader-Willi Syndrome
- D) Turner Syndrome

Answer:
B) Kallmann Syndrome

Explanation:
- Kallmann syndrome is a rare genetic disorder characterized by hypogonadotropic hypogonadism and anosmia. It results from a failure of GnRH neurons

to migrate during fetal development, leading to low levels of gonadotropins and sex hormones.

Pitfalls:

- Overlooking anosmia as part of the syndrome in the presence of other signs of hypogonadism.
- Misdiagnosing Kallmann syndrome as isolated hypogonadotropic hypogonadism.

Pearls:

- Treatment typically involves hormone replacement therapy (HRT), including testosterone for males.
- Genetic counseling is important, as the condition can be inherited in an X-linked recessive pattern.

Question 22:

Q: *A 58-year-old man with type 2 diabetes and obesity is not achieving glycemic control with metformin alone. Which of the following drugs offers additional weight loss benefits?*

- A) Metformin
- B) GLP-1 Receptor Agonists
- C) Insulin
- D) Thiazolidinediones

Answer:
B) GLP-1 Receptor Agonists
Explanation:

- GLP-1 receptor agonists (e.g., liraglutide, semaglutide) not only improve glycemic control but also promote weight loss and have cardiovascular benefits.

- These agents work by enhancing insulin secretion, inhibiting glucagon release, and promoting satiety.

Pitfalls:

- Misunderstanding the contraindications, such as a history of medullary thyroid cancer or pancreatitis.
- Overlooking the gastrointestinal side effects (nausea, vomiting) that are common with GLP-1 agonists.

Pearls:

- GLP-1 agonists should be considered early in patients with both diabetes and obesity, especially those at high cardiovascular risk.
- Monitor for adverse effects such as pancreatitis or gastrointestinal discomfort.

Question 23:

Q: A 50-year-old woman who recently underwent thyroidectomy presents with tetany, muscle cramps, and numbness around her lips. Serum calcium is 7 mg/dL (low), and phosphate is elevated. What is the first step in management?

- A) Oral Calcium and Vitamin D Supplements
- B) IV Calcium Gluconate
- C) Parathyroid Hormone Replacement
- D) Diuretics

Answer:

B) IV Calcium Gluconate

Explanation:

- The first step in managing acute hypocalcemia, especially in the setting of tetany and other symptoms, is intravenous calcium gluconate.
- Oral supplements are used for long-term management once the acute symptoms are controlled.

Pitfalls:
- Failing to recognize hypocalcemia in the post-thyroidectomy patient.
- Overcorrecting with calcium, which can lead to hypercalcemia and renal complications.

Pearls:
- Hypocalcemia should be managed cautiously, as rapid correction can cause complications like arrhythmias.
- Long-term management includes calcium and vitamin D supplementation.

Question 24:

Q: A 60-year-old hypertensive patient presents with paroxysmal headaches, sweating, and palpitations. Urinary catecholamine levels are elevated. What is the next step in the management of suspected pheochromocytoma?

- A) MRI of the Abdomen
- B) Abdominal Ultrasound
- C) 24-Hour Urinary Cortisol
- D) Preoperative Alpha-Blockade

Answer:
D) Preoperative Alpha-Blockade

Explanation:
- The next step in the management of pheochromocytoma is to initiate alpha-blockade (e.g., phenoxybenzamine) to control blood pressure before surgery.
- Beta-blockers are used after alpha-blockade to manage tachycardia.

Pitfalls:

- Starting beta-blockers before alpha-blockers, which can precipitate a hypertensive crisis.
- Overlooking the possibility of metastatic disease in patients with recurrent symptoms.

Pearls:

- Imaging (CT or MRI) of the adrenal glands follows the biochemical confirmation of pheochromocytoma.
- Surgical resection is the definitive treatment, with careful perioperative management to prevent hypertensive crises.

Question 25:

Q: A 30-year-old pregnant woman at 8 weeks gestation presents with fatigue and constipation. Her thyroid function test shows low TSH and normal free T4. What is the most likely diagnosis?

- A) Subclinical Hyperthyroidism
- B) Hypothyroidism
- C) Grave's Disease
- D) Pregnancy-Related Physiologic Changes

Answer:

A) Subclinical Hyperthyroidism

Explanation:

- During pregnancy, the increased levels of human chorionic gonadotropin (hCG) can lead to transient suppression of TSH.
- If free T4 is normal and TSH is mildly low, this is typically classified as subclinical hyperthyroidism, which is common during early pregnancy.

Pitfalls:

- Misinterpreting normal pregnancy-related changes in thyroid function as pathology.
- Failing to monitor thyroid function throughout pregnancy to avoid long-term complications.

Pearls:

- Regular monitoring of thyroid function is critical in pregnant women, as untreated thyroid disorders can adversely affect maternal and fetal health.
- If thyroid function worsens during pregnancy, treatment with thyroid hormone replacement should be considered.

Question 26:

Q: A 65-year-old woman presents with fatigue, polyuria, and kidney stones. Her serum calcium is elevated at 11.5 mg/dL, and parathyroid hormone (PTH) is also elevated. What is the next most appropriate diagnostic step?

- A) Urinary calcium excretion test
- B) CT scan of the abdomen
- C) Sestamibi scan of the parathyroid glands
- D) MRI of the neck

Answer:
C) Sestamibi scan of the parathyroid glands
Explanation:

- The diagnosis of primary hyperparathyroidism (PHPT) is confirmed with elevated calcium and PTH levels. A sestamibi scan (also known as a parathyroid scan) is used to localize the overactive parathyroid gland(s) prior to surgical resection.

- It is non-invasive and helps identify abnormal parathyroid tissue.

Pitfalls:
- Overlooking other causes of hypercalcemia (e.g., malignancy, granulomatous disease).
- Failing to consider secondary causes of hyperparathyroidism (e.g., chronic kidney disease).

Pearls:
- Surgical removal of the parathyroid adenoma is the definitive treatment for PHPT.
- Monitor kidney function and serum calcium levels after surgery to assess for normalization.

Question 27:

Q: *A 58-year-old man with a history of lung cancer presents with confusion, weakness, and a serum calcium level of 13.5 mg/dL. What is the most likely cause of his hypercalcemia?*

- A) Primary Hyperparathyroidism
- B) Metastatic Bone Disease
- C) Malignancy-Related Hypercalcemia (PTHrP-mediated)
- D) Vitamin D Toxicity

Answer:

C) Malignancy-Related Hypercalcemia (PTHrP-mediated)

Explanation:
- Hypercalcemia of malignancy is a common paraneoplastic syndrome, often mediated by parathyroid hormone-related peptide (PTHrP) produced by tumor cells. It typically occurs in advanced cancer, including lung and breast cancer.
- It is important to differentiate this from primary

hyperparathyroidism, which is less likely in patients with malignancy.

Pitfalls:

- Misinterpreting malignancy-related hypercalcemia as primary hyperparathyroidism.
- Failing to recognize the role of PTHrP in malignancy-related hypercalcemia.

Pearls:

- Immediate management includes hydration with normal saline and bisphosphonates (e.g., zoledronic acid) or denosumab to lower calcium levels.
- Correcting hypercalcemia can help improve symptoms of confusion and weakness.

Question 28:

Q: *A 72-year-old man with chronic kidney disease (CKD) presents with muscle cramps and bone pain. His serum calcium is low, phosphate is high, and PTH is markedly elevated. What is the most likely diagnosis?*

- A) Primary Hyperparathyroidism
- B) Vitamin D Deficiency
- C) Secondary Hyperparathyroidism
- D) Paget's Disease

Answer:

C) Secondary Hyperparathyroidism

Explanation:

- Secondary hyperparathyroidism is commonly seen in chronic kidney disease (CKD), where decreased renal function leads to phosphate retention and impaired activation of vitamin D, resulting in low calcium levels and compensatory high PTH.
- This form of hyperparathyroidism is different from

primary hyperparathyroidism, where PTH is elevated despite normal or high calcium levels.

Pitfalls:
- Failing to recognize that elevated PTH in CKD is compensatory rather than pathological.
- Overlooking the role of phosphate binders and vitamin D therapy in managing secondary hyperparathyroidism.

Pearls:
- Management involves controlling phosphate levels, correcting vitamin D deficiency, and considering the use of calcimimetics to suppress PTH.
- Early intervention can prevent bone disease and fractures associated with secondary hyperparathyroidism.

Question 29:

Q: *A 55-year-old female with long-standing chronic kidney disease (CKD) presents with bone pain and high calcium levels. Her PTH is also markedly elevated despite treatment for secondary hyperparathyroidism. What is the most likely diagnosis?*

- A) Primary Hyperparathyroidism
- B) Tertiary Hyperparathyroidism
- C) Hypercalcemia of Malignancy
- D) Vitamin D Intoxication

Answer:
B) Tertiary Hyperparathyroidism

Explanation:
- Tertiary hyperparathyroidism occurs when the parathyroid glands become autonomously hyperplastic and continue to overproduce PTH despite

correction of the underlying cause (such as chronic kidney disease). This results in both high calcium and elevated PTH levels.
- It typically occurs in long-standing CKD when there is prolonged stimulation of the parathyroid glands.

Pitfalls:
- Failing to differentiate tertiary hyperparathyroidism from primary hyperparathyroidism, where PTH is inappropriately elevated in the setting of normal or high calcium.
- Mismanagement of calcium levels without addressing the underlying parathyroid hyperplasia.

Pearls:
- Surgical removal of the hyperplastic parathyroid glands may be required in tertiary hyperparathyroidism.
- Regular monitoring of calcium and PTH levels in CKD patients is essential to prevent this complication.

Question 30:

Q: *A 62-year-old woman with a history of breast cancer presents with new-onset diarrhea, weight loss, and skin flushing. Serum cortisol and ACTH levels are low, and a CT scan reveals an adrenal mass. What paraneoplastic syndrome should you suspect?*
- A) Cushing's Syndrome
- B) Carcinoid Syndrome
- C) Hypercalcemia of Malignancy
- D) SIADH

Answer:

B) Carcinoid Syndrome

Explanation:
- Carcinoid syndrome is caused by neuroendocrine tumors (e.g., carcinoid tumors), often from the gastrointestinal tract or lungs, secreting serotonin and other vasoactive substances. It causes flushing, diarrhea, and wheezing.
- The association with breast cancer in this case may suggest a metastatic neuroendocrine tumor rather than a primary carcinoid tumor.

Pitfalls:
- Misattributing symptoms of flushing and diarrhea to other causes like menopause or medications.
- Failing to recognize carcinoid syndrome when only non-specific symptoms like diarrhea are present.

Pearls:
- Serotonin levels or urinary 5-HIAA may help confirm the diagnosis of carcinoid syndrome.
- Octreotide, a somatostatin analog, is the first-line treatment to manage symptoms and tumor growth.

Question 31:

Q: A 35-year-old woman presents with short stature, round face, and hoarseness. Her calcium is low, and PTH is elevated, but she is resistant to the effects of PTH. What is the most likely diagnosis?
- A) Primary Hyperparathyroidism
- B) Pseudohypoparathyroidism
- C) Secondary Hyperparathyroidism

- D) Hypoparathyroidism

Answer:

B) Pseudohypoparathyroidism

Explanation:

- Pseudohypoparathyroidism is a disorder characterized by resistance to PTH, despite elevated levels. It presents with hypocalcemia, elevated PTH, and features like short stature, obesity, and a round face.
- The condition is due to defects in the Gs alpha protein, leading to impaired signaling of PTH.

Pitfalls:

- Misdiagnosing pseudohypoparathyroidism as hypoparathyroidism, where both calcium and PTH are low.
- Failing to recognize the characteristic physical features of the disorder.

Pearls:

- Genetic testing is often needed to confirm pseudohypoparathyroidism.
- Treatment involves calcium and vitamin D supplementation, though the response can be variable.

Question 32:

Q: *A 42-year-old woman with known Addison's disease presents with severe hypotension, vomiting, and confusion. Her serum sodium is 128 mmol/L, potassium is 6.2 mmol/L, and glucose is 45 mg/dL. What is the most immediate treatment?*

- A) Oral glucose tablets
- B) Intravenous corticosteroids

- C) Intravenous fluids with dextrose
- D) Calcium gluconate infusion

Answer:

B) Intravenous corticosteroids

Explanation:

- Acute adrenal insufficiency, or Addisonian crisis, is a medical emergency requiring immediate administration of **intravenous corticosteroids**, such as hydrocortisone, to replace deficient cortisol.
- This crisis is often precipitated by stressors like infection or trauma and leads to hypotension, hyponatremia, hyperkalemia, and hypoglycemia.
- IV fluids (saline) and glucose are important adjuncts to correct dehydration and hypoglycemia, but the primary treatment is corticosteroid replacement.

Pitfalls:

- Delaying corticosteroid administration while focusing on other symptoms like hypoglycemia.
- Misdiagnosing acute adrenal insufficiency as septic shock or other causes of hypotension.

Pearls:

- Always consider **Addisonian crisis** in any patient with known adrenal insufficiency who presents with severe hypotension, confusion, or gastrointestinal symptoms, particularly during periods of stress.
- IV hydrocortisone (100 mg) should be given promptly in emergencies, followed by continuous infusion or repeat doses as needed.

Question 33:

Q: *A 55-year-old male with unexplained weight loss, fatigue, and salt cravings is found to have low morning serum cortisol levels. A low-dose ACTH stimulation test shows poor cortisol response. What is the next step in managing this patient?*

- A) Initiate high-dose glucocorticoid therapy
- B) Perform an MRI of the adrenal glands
- C) Check for adrenal antibodies
- D) Start fludrocortisone therapy

Answer:
C) Check for adrenal antibodies

Explanation:

- **Addison's disease** is characterized by primary adrenal insufficiency, often due to autoimmune destruction of the adrenal glands. The diagnosis is confirmed by a **poor response to the ACTH stimulation test** (or a low baseline cortisol level).
- **Adrenal antibodies** (e.g., 21-hydroxylase antibodies) can help confirm autoimmune Addison's disease.
- MRI of the adrenal glands is not typically performed first unless there is concern for an adrenal tumor or hemorrhage.

Pitfalls:

- Failing to consider other causes of adrenal insufficiency, such as **pituitary dysfunction** (secondary adrenal insufficiency).
- Starting therapy without confirming the etiology of the adrenal insufficiency.

Pearls:

- **Adrenal antibodies** are a key diagnostic test in autoimmune Addison's disease.
- Treatment for Addison's disease involves both glucocorticoids (hydrocortisone) and mineralocorticoids (fludrocortisone), and it should be lifelong.

Question 34:

Q: *A 60-year-old man on chronic prednisone therapy for rheumatoid arthritis presents with weakness, fever, and hypotension. His serum sodium is 132 mmol/L, potassium is 5.4 mmol/L, and blood glucose is 50 mg/dL. What is the most likely diagnosis?*
- A) Adrenal crisis due to abrupt steroid withdrawal
- B) Septic shock
- C) Diabetic ketoacidosis
- D) Acute myocardial infarction

Answer:
A) Adrenal crisis due to abrupt steroid withdrawal

Explanation:
- Patients on long-term **glucocorticoid therapy**, like prednisone, are at risk for **adrenal insufficiency** due to suppression of the hypothalamic-pituitary-adrenal axis.
- Abrupt withdrawal of steroids or inadequate stress dosing in these patients can precipitate an **adrenal crisis**, characterized by hypotension, hyponatremia, hyperkalemia, and hypoglycemia.
- Treatment involves urgent **glucocorticoid replacement** (IV hydrocortisone) and supportive care.

Pitfalls:
- Failing to recognize adrenal crisis in patients on

chronic steroid therapy.
- Confusing adrenal crisis with sepsis or other causes of hypotension.

Pearls:
- Patients on long-term steroid therapy should be **tapered off** gradually to allow adrenal recovery.
- During acute illness or surgery, **stress doses** of corticosteroids are required to prevent adrenal crisis.

Question 35:

Q: A 38-year-old woman with a history of Cushing's syndrome presents with vomiting, hypotension, and confusion after undergoing a recent surgery. Her serum cortisol is low despite ACTH administration. What is the most likely cause of her symptoms?

- A) Adrenal crisis due to steroid withdrawal
- B) Sepsis
- C) Acute myocardial infarction
- D) Acute renal failure

Answer:
A) Adrenal crisis due to steroid withdrawal

Explanation:

- **Cushing's syndrome** results in hypercortisolism, often due to long-term steroid use or an adrenal tumor. After treatment (such as surgery or adrenalectomy), patients can experience **adrenal insufficiency** due to suppression of the adrenal glands.
- In this case, the low cortisol level despite ACTH stimulation suggests **adrenal crisis** following steroid withdrawal.
- Treatment includes IV hydrocortisone and supportive care for shock.

Pitfalls:

- Misdiagnosing adrenal crisis as septic shock or another complication of surgery.
- Failing to provide appropriate glucocorticoid replacement in patients with a history of Cushing's syndrome.

Pearls:

- **Stress dosing** of glucocorticoids is essential for patients who have undergone treatment for Cushing's syndrome, especially after surgery or in cases of acute illness.
- Gradual tapering off steroids is crucial to prevent adrenal insufficiency.

Question 36:

Q: *A 45-year-old woman with known Addison's disease presents with weakness, nausea, and palpitations. Her serum potassium is 6.9 mmol/L, sodium is 132 mmol/L, and chloride is low. What is the most likely explanation for her hyperkalemia?*

- A) Acute kidney injury
- B) Addison's disease and mineralocorticoid deficiency
- C) Diabetic ketoacidosis
- D) Hyperaldosteronism

Answer:

B) Addison's disease and mineralocorticoid deficiency

Explanation:

- Hyperkalemia in **Addison's disease** is typically caused by **mineralocorticoid deficiency**, specifically a lack of aldosterone, which normally promotes sodium reabsorption and potassium excretion in the kidneys.
- In the absence of adequate aldosterone, potassium retention occurs, leading to elevated serum potassium levels.

Pitfalls:

- Misdiagnosing hyperkalemia as a result of other conditions like **acute kidney injury** without considering the patient's history of Addison's disease.

- Overlooking the need for **mineralocorticoid therapy** (fludrocortisone) in the treatment of Addison's disease.

Pearls:

- **Fludrocortisone** is critical in treating the **mineralocorticoid deficiency** in Addison's disease and should be carefully adjusted based on clinical response and electrolyte levels.
- Close monitoring of **electrolytes** (particularly potassium) is required in patients with Addison's disease.

Question 37:

Q: A 55-year-old man with Type 2 diabetes presents with confusion and sweating. His blood glucose is 45 mg/dL. What is the first step in management?

- A) Administer 50 mL of 50% dextrose IV
- B) Administer 1 mg glucagon IM
- C) Administer insulin
- D) Provide oral glucose if the patient is conscious

Answer:
D) Provide oral glucose if the patient is conscious

Explanation:

- For conscious patients with **mild to moderate hypoglycemia**, oral glucose is the first-line treatment. This can be in the form of glucose tablets, juice, or regular soda.
- If the patient is unconscious, IV dextrose (50%) or glucagon (IM) should be used, depending on the available resources and setting.

Pitfalls:

- Administering IV dextrose when the patient is conscious, which is unnecessary and might complicate management.
- Delaying treatment or underestimating the severity of hypoglycemia.

Pearls:

- **Rapid-acting carbohydrate** (e.g., glucose or juice) is the fastest and most effective way to treat hypoglycemia in conscious patients.
- Monitor blood glucose levels regularly after treatment

to ensure it has normalized.

Question 38:

Q: *A 32-year-old woman in her first trimester presents with fatigue, constipation, and weight gain. Her thyroid function tests show a TSH of 5.9 µU/mL (normal range: 0.4-4.0), free T4 of 0.8 ng/dL (normal range: 0.9-1.7), and normal free T3. What is the most appropriate management?*

- A) Initiate levothyroxine therapy
- B) No treatment; repeat thyroid function tests after pregnancy
- C) Increase iodine supplementation
- D) Refer for thyroid biopsy

Answer:

A) Initiate levothyroxine therapy

Explanation:

- The patient has **subclinical hypothyroidism**, characterized by elevated TSH with normal free T4. In pregnancy, particularly in the first trimester, thyroid function is crucial for fetal development.
- **Hypothyroidism in pregnancy** can be associated with poor pregnancy outcomes, such as preterm birth and developmental delays. **Levothyroxine** is the treatment of choice to maintain thyroid function within the normal range.

Pitfalls:

- Misdiagnosing subclinical hypothyroidism as normal pregnancy changes, leading to delayed treatment.
- Failing to adjust levothyroxine dosage based on trimester-specific requirements during pregnancy.

Pearls:

- **Thyroid dysfunction** in pregnancy should be closely monitored, as maternal hypothyroidism can affect fetal development, particularly brain development.
- **Levothyroxine** should be adjusted to achieve a target TSH of <2.5 µU/mL in the first trimester.

Question 39:

Q: *A 28-year-old woman at 10 weeks of gestation presents with palpitations, heat intolerance, and weight loss. Her thyroid function tests show low TSH (<0.01 µU/mL), high free T4, and normal free T3. What is the most likely diagnosis, and what is the best treatment option?*

- A) Graves' disease; treat with propylthiouracil (PTU)
- B) Hyperemesis gravidarum; treat with antiemetics
- C) Subacute thyroiditis; treat with NSAIDs
- D) Toxic multinodular goiter; treat with radioactive iodine

Answer:
A) Graves' disease; treat with propylthiouracil (PTU)
Explanation:
- The patient presents with **hyperthyroidism** in pregnancy, most likely due to **Graves' disease**. In pregnancy, **Graves' disease** should be managed carefully with antithyroid drugs, as untreated hyperthyroidism can lead to preterm labor, low birth weight, and fetal thyroid dysfunction.
- **Propylthiouracil (PTU)** is preferred in the first trimester due to a lower risk of teratogenic effects compared to methimazole.

Pitfalls:
- Using methimazole, which is contraindicated during

the first trimester due to teratogenicity.
- Overlooking the need for close monitoring of maternal thyroid function and fetal growth.

Pearls:
- **Propylthiouracil** (PTU) is used in the first trimester for **Graves' disease**, but can be switched to methimazole after the first trimester.
- Regular monitoring of **fetal thyroid function** is important during the treatment of hyperthyroidism in pregnancy.

Question 40:

Q: A 6-year-old child presents with irritability, weight loss despite a good appetite, and a goiter. His thyroid function tests show low TSH and elevated free T4. What is the most likely diagnosis, and how should it be treated?
- A) Hashimoto's thyroiditis; treat with levothyroxine
- B) Graves' disease; treat with antithyroid medication
- C) Toxic multinodular goiter; treat with radioactive iodine
- D) Subclinical hyperthyroidism; monitor only

Answer:
B) Graves' disease; treat with antithyroid medication

Explanation:
- In children, **Graves' disease** is the most common cause of hyperthyroidism. The elevated T4 with low TSH, along with symptoms like irritability and weight loss despite increased appetite, is characteristic.
- **Antithyroid medications**, such as **methimazole** or **propylthiouracil**, are used as the first-line treatment. If medical therapy fails, radioactive iodine therapy or

surgery may be considered.

Pitfalls:

- Failing to differentiate between **Graves' disease** and other causes of thyroid dysfunction in children, such as thyroiditis or autoimmune thyroid diseases.
- Delaying treatment of hyperthyroidism in children, which can lead to serious complications like growth failure or bone loss.

Pearls:

- **Graves' disease** is the most common cause of hyperthyroidism in children and should be managed with antithyroid drugs to avoid complications.
- Close monitoring of growth and development is critical in pediatric patients with thyroid disorders.

Question 41:

Q: *A 72-year-old woman presents with fatigue, cold intolerance, and constipation. Her thyroid function tests show a TSH of 8.5 µU/mL, free T4 of 0.6 ng/dL, and normal free T3. What is the best initial approach to treatment in this elderly patient?*

- A) Start high-dose levothyroxine therapy
- B) Initiate low-dose levothyroxine and titrate upwards
- C) No treatment needed; repeat thyroid function tests in 6 months
- D) Refer for thyroidectomy

Answer:

B) Initiate low-dose levothyroxine and titrate upwards

Explanation:

- **Elderly patients** with hypothyroidism should be treated cautiously with **low-dose levothyroxine** and gradually increased to avoid complications like

arrhythmias.
- Start with a low dose (e.g., 25-50 µg/day) and titrate upward based on the patient's response and thyroid function tests. High doses of levothyroxine can precipitate **cardiac events** (e.g., atrial fibrillation) in the elderly.

Pitfalls:
- Starting at too high of a dose, leading to exacerbation of cardiovascular risks in elderly patients.
- Assuming that all elderly patients with mildly elevated TSH need immediate treatment without considering other possible causes of symptoms.

Pearls:
- **Levothyroxine** should be started at lower doses in the elderly to avoid exacerbating underlying cardiac conditions.
- Monitor for signs of over-replacement, such as **atrial fibrillation** or **osteoporosis**, particularly in elderly women.

Question 42:

Q: *A 30-year-old pregnant woman at 24 weeks of gestation is diagnosed with gestational diabetes mellitus (GDM) after a 75g oral glucose tolerance test (OGTT) shows a fasting glucose of 110 mg/dL, 1-hour glucose of 180 mg/dL, and 2-hour glucose of 160 mg/dL. What is the most appropriate next step in management?*
- A) Start insulin therapy immediately
- B) Start metformin therapy
- C) Begin lifestyle modifications, including diet and exercise
- D) Perform a repeat OGTT at 28 weeks

Answer:

C) Begin lifestyle modifications, including diet and exercise

Explanation:

- **Gestational diabetes mellitus (GDM)** is diagnosed based on elevated glucose levels in pregnancy, and **lifestyle modification** (diet and exercise) is the first-line treatment.
- If blood glucose levels remain elevated despite these interventions, **insulin** therapy or **metformin** may be initiated.

Pitfalls:

- Delaying the initiation of lifestyle modifications or insulin therapy, which could worsen the pregnancy outcome.
- Misdiagnosing gestational diabetes as a normal pregnancy-related change in glucose metabolism.

Pearls:

- Tight glucose control during pregnancy is crucial to reduce the risk of maternal and fetal complications, including macrosomia and preterm labor.
- **Insulin therapy** is safe during pregnancy and is preferred if lifestyle changes alone are insufficient.

Question 43:

Q: *A 28-year-old pregnant woman presents with hypercalcemia and mild hypertension during her second trimester. Her calcium levels are 11.2 mg/dL (normal range: 8.5-10.2), and parathyroid hormone (PTH) is elevated. What is the most likely diagnosis?*

- A) Primary hyperparathyroidism
- B) Gestational hypercalcemia
- C) Vitamin D toxicity
- D) Preeclampsia

Answer:

A) Primary hyperparathyroidism

Explanation:

- **Primary hyperparathyroidism** (PHPT) during pregnancy is uncommon but can lead to **hypercalcemia** and an elevated **PTH** level.
- This condition can lead to serious maternal and fetal complications, including preeclampsia and fetal skeletal abnormalities. Surgical treatment may be necessary if medical management does not control symptoms.

Pitfalls:

- Failing to identify **primary hyperparathyroidism** in the context of pregnancy and mistakenly attributing the symptoms to more common pregnancy-related issues like preeclampsia.
- Overlooking the need for surgical intervention in severe cases of hypercalcemia during pregnancy.

Pearls:

- Pregnant women with **primary hyperparathyroidism** should be carefully monitored for maternal and fetal health, and surgery is often recommended if the condition is severe.
- **Medical management** may include hydration and calcium-lowering agents until surgical intervention can be performed safely.

Question 44:

Q: *A 45-year-old woman presents with palpitations, heat intolerance, weight loss, and anxiety. Her TSH is undetectable, and her free T4 is elevated. The radioiodine uptake scan shows diffuse uptake throughout the thyroid gland. What is the most likely diagnosis, and what is the next step in management?*

- A) Graves' disease; initiate methimazole therapy
- B) Toxic multinodular goiter; initiate radioactive iodine therapy
- C) Subacute thyroiditis; start NSAIDs
- D) Thyroid storm; administer beta-blockers and hydrocortisone

Answer:
A) Graves' disease; initiate methimazole therapy

Explanation:

- The combination of **undetectable TSH, elevated free T4**, and **diffuse radioactive iodine uptake** suggests **Graves' disease**, an autoimmune disorder causing hyperthyroidism.
- First-line treatment for Graves' disease includes **methimazole** or **propylthiouracil (PTU)** (especially in pregnancy), to inhibit thyroid hormone synthesis.
- **Radioactive iodine therapy** is an option for definitive treatment if medical therapy fails or is not well tolerated.

Pitfalls:

- Misdiagnosing **Graves' disease** as **toxic multinodular goiter** or **subacute thyroiditis**, as the clinical presentation can overlap.
- Not recognizing the need for **beta-blockers** to manage symptoms (e.g., palpitations and tremors) in the acute

phase.

Pearls:

- **Methimazole** is preferred in the treatment of Graves' disease, but **PTU** is recommended in the first trimester of pregnancy.
- **Radioactive iodine therapy** is usually reserved for patients who do not respond to antithyroid drugs or have recurrent disease.

Question 45:

Q: *A 50-year-old male presents with central obesity, purple striae, hypertension, and easy bruising. His serum cortisol is elevated. A dexamethasone suppression test is performed, and there is no suppression of cortisol. What is the next diagnostic step?*

- A) ACTH level measurement
- B) MRI of the pituitary
- C) Abdominal CT to assess for adrenal adenoma
- D) 24-hour urinary cortisol measurement

Answer:

A) ACTH level measurement

Explanation:

- The clinical presentation is highly suggestive of **Cushing's syndrome**, which is characterized by excess cortisol. The **lack of suppression** on the dexamethasone test suggests **ACTH-dependent Cushing's syndrome**, which is usually caused by a pituitary adenoma (Cushing's disease) or ectopic ACTH production.
- The first diagnostic step is to measure **ACTH levels** to distinguish between **ACTH-dependent** and **ACTH-independent** causes (e.g., adrenal adenoma).

- If ACTH is low, the source is likely an adrenal tumor, and imaging such as **abdominal CT** would be appropriate.

Pitfalls:

- Failing to measure **ACTH** levels early in the diagnostic process and jumping directly to imaging studies without proper differentiation between pituitary and adrenal causes.
- Misinterpreting the absence of suppression on the dexamethasone test as a definitive diagnosis without further confirming the source of excess cortisol.

Pearls:

- A high **ACTH level** points towards a **pituitary adenoma** or ectopic ACTH production, while a low **ACTH** suggests an **adrenal source**.
- **MRI of the pituitary** is the next step if ACTH levels are elevated and Cushing's disease is suspected.

Question 46:

Q: *A 40-year-old woman with uncontrolled hypertension despite multiple antihypertensive medications presents with hypokalemia. Her plasma aldosterone concentration is elevated, and the plasma renin activity is suppressed. What is the next appropriate diagnostic step?*

- A) CT scan of the adrenal glands
- B) Adrenal vein sampling
- C) Serum ACTH levels
- D) Genetic testing for familial hyperaldosteronism

Answer:
B) Adrenal vein sampling

Explanation:
- This patient exhibits signs of **primary hyperaldosteronism** (also known as Conn's syndrome), characterized by **hypertension, hypokalemia**, and elevated aldosterone with suppressed renin.
- The next step in the diagnosis is **adrenal vein sampling**, which can help differentiate between a **unilateral adrenal adenoma** and **bilateral adrenal hyperplasia**, guiding further treatment options.
- If an adenoma is found, surgical removal is often the treatment, whereas bilateral hyperplasia is managed medically with aldosterone antagonists like **spironolactone**.

Pitfalls:
- Relying solely on imaging studies, like CT scans, without confirming the diagnosis via **adrenal vein sampling** can lead to false positives or incorrect treatment decisions.
- Misinterpreting **secondary causes of hyperaldosteronism** as primary due to incorrect labeling of the patient's renin-aldosterone ratio.

Pearls:
- **Adrenal vein sampling** is essential for confirming the source of aldosterone excess, particularly when planning for surgery.
- **Spironolactone** is a key treatment for **bilateral adrenal hyperplasia**, while **unilateral adrenal adenomas** may require surgical resection.

Question 47:

Q: *A 38-year-old man presents with gradual enlargement of his hands and feet, facial changes (e.g., protruding jaw), and excessive sweating. His serum IGF-1 levels are elevated. What is the next step in the diagnosis?*

- A) MRI of the pituitary
- B) Oral glucose tolerance test (OGTT)
- C) Serum cortisol test
- D) Measurement of serum prolactin

Answer:
A) MRI of the pituitary

Explanation:

- **Acromegaly** is most commonly caused by a **pituitary adenoma** secreting growth hormone (GH). The elevated **IGF-1** is a marker of excess growth hormone secretion.
- An **MRI of the pituitary** is the next step to visualize the pituitary gland and confirm the presence of a tumor.
- An **OGTT** may be used to confirm acromegaly by demonstrating an inability to suppress GH after glucose intake, but **MRI** is the gold standard for identifying the tumor.

Pitfalls:

- Failing to consider acromegaly in patients with **gradual changes** in physical appearance or nonspecific symptoms.
- Not performing an **MRI** if IGF-1 levels are elevated,

leading to missed diagnoses of pituitary adenomas.

Pearls:

- In **acromegaly**, IGF-1 levels are usually more reliable than GH measurements for diagnosis.
- **MRI** is the gold standard for detecting **pituitary adenomas**, which are the most common cause of acromegaly.

Question 48:

Q: *A 60-year-old man with a history of **Addison's disease** presents with fever, confusion, and hypotension after missing several doses of his corticosteroid medication. His sodium is low, and potassium is high. What is the most appropriate next step in treatment?*

- A) Increase the dose of oral prednisone
- B) Administer intravenous hydrocortisone
- C) Start a dopamine infusion
- D) Administer oral salt tablets

Answer:

B) Administer intravenous hydrocortisone

Explanation:

- This patient is experiencing an **adrenal crisis**, a life-threatening condition that occurs in individuals with **Addison's disease** when there is insufficient cortisol production, usually triggered by infection, stress, or missed steroid doses.
- The immediate treatment is **IV hydrocortisone**, along with **fluid resuscitation** and electrolyte correction.
- **Hydrocortisone** is preferred over prednisone in crisis situations due to its potent glucocorticoid effects.

Pitfalls:

- Misdiagnosing **adrenal crisis** as sepsis or another

infectious cause, which may delay the administration of essential corticosteroid therapy.
- Failing to provide appropriate fluid resuscitation and electrolyte correction, which are critical components of treatment.

Pearls:

- **Adrenal crisis** is a medical emergency requiring prompt administration of **IV hydrocortisone**, **fluid resuscitation**, and electrolyte management.
- Patients with **Addison's disease** should be educated on stress dosing during illness and how to manage missed steroid doses.

Question 49:

Q: A 45-year-old woman presents with uncontrolled hypertension despite being on a combination of antihypertensive medications. She also reports muscle weakness, frequent urination, and headaches. Her potassium level is 2.9 mEq/L, and her serum sodium is normal. A plasma aldosterone concentration is 1200 ng/dL, and the plasma renin activity is suppressed. What is the most likely diagnosis, and what is the next best step in management?

- A) Primary hyperaldosteronism (Conn's syndrome); perform adrenal vein sampling
- B) Secondary hyperaldosteronism due to renovascular disease; obtain an abdominal CT angiogram
- C) Pheochromocytoma; perform urinary catecholamine analysis
- D) Hyperthyroidism; assess thyroid function tests

Answer:
A) Primary hyperaldosteronism (Conn's syndrome); perform adrenal vein sampling

Explanation:
- The patient's **hypokalemia**, **hypertension**, and suppressed **plasma renin activity** are classic signs of **primary hyperaldosteronism** (Conn's syndrome), which is characterized by excessive aldosterone production from the adrenal glands.
- The next step in management is **adrenal vein sampling** to differentiate between **unilateral adrenal adenoma** (which can be treated with surgery) and **bilateral adrenal hyperplasia** (treated medically with **spironolactone** or **eplerenone**).
- **Adrenal vein sampling** is the gold standard for localizing the source of aldosterone excess.

Pitfalls:
- Misdiagnosing **primary hyperaldosteronism** as secondary hypertension, especially in patients with other causes of electrolyte disturbances, without performing the necessary diagnostic tests.
- Jumping directly to **CT imaging** of the adrenal glands without proper confirmation through **adrenal vein sampling** can lead to inappropriate treatment plans.

Pearls:
- A **low potassium level**, **hypertension**, and **low renin levels** suggest **primary hyperaldosteronism**.
- **Adrenal vein sampling** is crucial for confirming unilateral versus bilateral adrenal involvement before deciding on surgery or medical management.

Question 50:

Q: *A 52-year-old man is diagnosed with **primary hyperaldosteronism (Conn's syndrome)** based on elevated aldosterone levels and suppressed renin activity. Imaging reveals a unilateral adrenal adenoma. What is the most appropriate treatment for this patient?*

- A) Spironolactone therapy
- B) Surgery: adrenalectomy
- C) Radiofrequency ablation of the adrenal gland
- D) Start a thiazide diuretic for blood pressure control

Answer:
B) Surgery: adrenalectomy

Explanation:

- In patients with **primary hyperaldosteronism** due to a **unilateral adrenal adenoma**, the most appropriate treatment is **adrenalectomy**, which can cure the condition by removing the adenoma and halting the excess aldosterone production.
- While **spironolactone** or **eplerenone** can be used as medical management, especially for **bilateral adrenal hyperplasia**, **adrenalectomy** is the definitive treatment for **unilateral adenomas**.
- **Spironolactone** may be used temporarily for blood pressure and potassium control before surgery or in patients with **bilateral adrenal hyperplasia**.

Pitfalls:

- Delaying surgery in patients with **unilateral adrenal adenomas**, potentially leading to prolonged hypertension and electrolyte disturbances.
- Misinterpreting **bilateral adrenal hyperplasia** as an indication for surgery instead of medical management with aldosterone antagonists like **spironolactone**.

Pearls:

- **Unilateral adrenal adenomas** causing **primary hyperaldosteronism** should be treated with **adrenalectomy** for long-term resolution.
- **Spironolactone** or **eplerenone** is effective for patients with **bilateral adrenal hyperplasia** but not for unilateral adenomas.
- Postoperative monitoring of blood pressure and electrolytes is essential after **adrenalectomy**.

www.ingramcontent.com/pod-product-compliance
Lightning Source LLC
Chambersburg PA
CBHW071653240526
45469CB00021B/2278